Ice Bucket Challenge:

What it means for ALS and Lou Gehrig's disease.

Introduction

I want to thank you and congratulate you for downloading the book, "*Ice Bucket Challenge*".

This book contains information on what the Ice Bucket Challenge is and what it is accomplishing.

Thanks again for downloading this book, I hope you enjoy it!

This document is geared towards providing exact and reliable information in regards to the topic and issue covered. The publication is sold with the idea that the publisher is not required to render accounting, officially permitted, or otherwise, qualified services. If advice is necessary, legal or professional, a practiced individual in the profession should be ordered.

The information provided herein is stated to be truthful and consistent, in that any liability, in terms

Chapter 1: A cold bucket of water

We've all seen the videos. Everyone from your favorite celebrity to people you know from all walks of life are taking a bucket of cold water and ice and dumping it over their heads. In fact there's a good chance you may be even called out tomorrow to take part in the ice bucket challenge yourself! What does it all mean? What is ALS and Lou Gehrig's disease? This book will give you an overview of what the Ice Bucket Challenge has done for people with ALS across the nation.

The premise is simple. You've been called out by a friend. You must either be filmed having a bucket of frigid ice water dumped over your head or donate $100 to an ALS charity of your choice. Some people even do both these challenges. Lastly, the person then calls out 3 of their friends to next take part in the ice bucket challenge. The whole spectacle is usually filmed and uploaded to a social medial outlet where it then continues to spread like wildfire. It seems as if everyone is taking part in this from movie stars to ex-presidents to country singers.

It started out as a challenge from golfer Chris Kennedy to his cousin in New York. That cousin's husband is one who has battled ALS or Lou Gehrig's disease for 11 years. Soon after that video was posted, Pete Frates, Boston College star and ALS diagnosed patient, shared the video on his social media pages and the rest was history in the making.

Chapter 2: What is ALS?

ALS, or Lou Gehrig's disease as it is sometimes called, is a neurodegenerative disease with no cure known so far. Its full name is "amyotrophic lateral sclerosis". Most people do not know someone with ALS but you may recognize the name Stephen Hawking. Dr. Hawking is one of the greatest minds of our time and also a diagnosed patient of ALS.

The disease was first discovered in 1869 by Jean-Martin Charcot. Charcot was a neurologist who studied medicine in Paris, France. Most people however attribute ALS with the legendary baseball player, Lou Gehrig. The eye of the nation was on Gehrig as he was one of the best baseball players in the year

1939. It was only then that the world really started to see what ALS was and how it would effect a person diagnosed with the disease.

ALS effects the diagnosed in many different ways. The muscles become stiffened.Weakness travels through the subject as a result of the atrophy of the muscles. It becomes increasingly more and more difficult for the patient to talk and most people will need the help of a device in order to communicate. It makes breathing and swallowing nearly impossible as well.

There is currently no absolute diagnosis as to why ALS occurs. The treatment is more for the symptoms and not for the diseases itself. Physical therapy is included in the regimen of the patient as well to help with the limbering out of the muscles and to increase the strength of the patient.

Chapter 3: Is an ice bucket really doing anything?

There have been an increasing number of critics of the ice bucket challenge. The concerns are that most people seem to not even be aware of what the disease is and are just participating in order to become popular again for a few minutes on Facebook or the news.

There may be some truth to this but let's look at the facts for a minute. Since the challenge started not so many months ago in mid 2014 to late August of the same year, the ALS Association has seen donations rise up to almost 16 million dollars total. This amount is almost 10 times the amount of what would normally come in for donations during that time. You can't argue with the numbers like that. The ice bucket challenge has changed our world for the better.

It's good for a number of reasons. People are talking about the disease more than ever now and wondering what it is and what they can do to help. It's ok to be entertained as long as we also follow through with the support, the education, and helping those that need to be helped. Our world is constantly bombarded with depressing news and when we are able to see our favorite relative or celebrity take part in helping out a disease that is ok and should be inspiring to us all.

Chapter 4: What can I do?

You may be asking yourself "What can I do to help?". Here are some things you can do. First you must be aware of the facts. Know what ALS is and know what the myths are about this horrible disease as well.

Visit websites like www.alsa.org to find out current information and support groups or chapters in your state. Sign up to be involved with a Walk to Defeat ALS walk to help raise more money for ALS research. Inquire about volunteering at local hospitals and nursing homes to see if there are ways that you can help those with ALS in a one on one environment.

Eventually the ice bucket challenge videos will stop. It is our job to not let the ice melt away in our memories but to keep the fight alive for defeating ALS once and for all. The ice bucket challenge has united our curiosity as a nation. Let's challenge ourselves and those we love around us to make a difference today.

Conclusion

Thank you again for downloading this book!

I hope this book was able to help you to give you some pertinent information regarding ALS and the ice bucket challenge.

The next step is to get involved in your local community raising awareness for ALS.

Finally, if you enjoyed this book, then I'd like to ask you for a favor, would you be kind enough to leave a review for this book on Amazon? It'd be greatly appreciated!

Thank you and good luck!

www.ingramcontent.com/pod-product-compliance
Lightning Source LLC
Chambersburg PA
CBHW062033280526
45787CB00005B/2308